TYPE 2 DIA

Food List

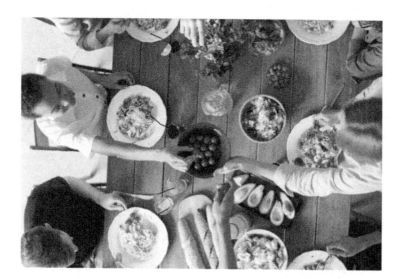

Empower Yourself with Diabetes-Friendly
Foods and Expert Meal Planning
Guidance for Optimal Health

BELL QUINTANA

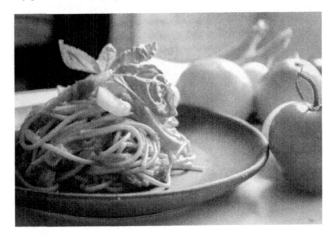

TABLE OF CONTENT

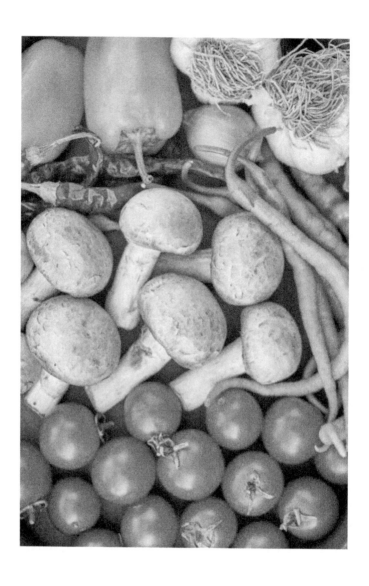

Share Your Experience with 'Type 2 Diabetes Food List'"

Thank you for choosing 'Type 2 Diabetes Food List'!

If you find this book helpful and insightful on your journey to better diabetes management, we kindly ask you to consider leaving a review on Amazon.

Your valuable feedback will not only inspire others but also motivate us to continue providing valuable content to support your health goals. Happy reading and thank you for being part of our community!

INTRODUCTION

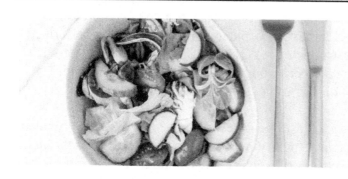

Welcome to "Type 2 Diabetes Food List," your comprehensive guide to managing Type 2 diabetes through a balanced and diabetes-friendly diet. If you or a loved one have been diagnosed with Type 2 diabetes, you know how crucial it is to maintain stable blood sugar levels to lead a healthy and fulfilling life. This book aims to equip you with the knowledge and practical tips to make informed food choices, create delicious and nutritious meals, and embrace a lifestyle that supports your diabetes management journey.

Living with Type 2 diabetes can be overwhelming, and the abundance of conflicting information about dietary choices can make it even more challenging to know where to start. However, with the right guidance and understanding of how food affects your blood sugar, you can take charge of your health and prevent the complications associated with diabetes.

Now, let me share a story that illustrates the impact of adopting a Type 2 diabetes-friendly diet and how it transformed the life of John, a man who faced the challenges of managing his condition.

John's journey with diabetes began with feelings of confusion and uncertainty. He struggled to control his blood sugar levels despite taking medication as prescribed. With each doctor's visit, his frustration grew, and he couldn't help but wonder if there was a way to regain control of his health.

One day, a close friend recommended a book that provided invaluable insights into managing Type 2 diabetes through dietary changes. Skeptical but willing to try anything, John decided to give it a shot. As he delved into the pages of "Type 2 Diabetes Food List," he discovered a wealth of information about the impact of different foods on blood sugar levels.

The book's practical guidance and easy-to-follow food lists empowered John to make smarter choices when planning his meals. He learned to focus on nutrient-dense foods, like non-starchy vegetables, lean proteins, and healthy fats, while avoiding sugary and processed items. Armed with this newfound knowledge, John ventured into the world of cooking and experimented with recipes that catered to his dietary needs.

As the weeks passed, John noticed remarkable changes. His blood sugar levels began to stabilize, and his energy levels increased. The constant feelings of fatigue and mood swings diminished. The more he embraced the guidelines from the book, the more confident he became in managing his diabetes.

Months later, during a routine check-up, John's doctor was astonished by the improvement in his overall health. His A1C levels had dropped significantly, and his need for medication reduced. The doctor praised John's commitment to his diet and lifestyle changes, emphasizing how vital they were in controlling his condition effectively.

John's story is just one of many examples of how a well-informed approach to eating can positively impact the lives of those living with Type 2 diabetes. With dedication and determination, you too can achieve better blood sugar control, enhanced overall health, and a brighter future.

This book is here to support you on your journey, providing a clear and concise roadmap to navigate the complex world of food choices, meal planning, and diabetes management. It is our hope that, armed with this knowledge, you will discover the power you hold to make transformative changes in your life and embrace a happier, healthier tomorrow. Let's get started!

CHAPTER 1

THE BASICS OF A TYPE 2 DIABETES-FRIENDLY DIET

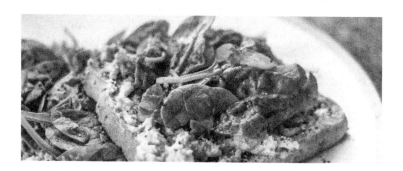

Living with Type 2 diabetes requires a thoughtful and strategic approach to your diet. In this chapter, we will explore the fundamentals of a Type 2 diabetes-friendly diet, focusing on how carbohydrates, proteins, fats, portion control, and meal timing can play crucial roles in managing your blood sugar levels.

CARBOHYDRATES AND BLOOD SUGAR

Carbohydrates have the most significant impact on blood sugar levels, as they break down into glucose during digestion. This glucose then enters the bloodstream, leading to spikes in blood sugar levels. It is essential to be mindful of the type and quantity of carbohydrates you consume.

- **Understanding Glycemic Index (GI):** The glycemic index ranks carbohydrates based on how quickly they raise blood sugar levels. Low-GI foods, such as whole grains, legumes, and non-starchy vegetables, cause a slower and more gradual increase in blood sugar, promoting better glucose control.

- **Focus on Fiber:** Foods rich in dietary fiber can slow down the absorption of glucose and help maintain stable blood sugar levels. Incorporating whole grains, fruits, vegetables, and nuts into your diet can provide valuable fiber.

- **Limiting High-Glycemic Foods:** Foods with a high GI, like sugary snacks, refined grains, and sweetened beverages, should be consumed in moderation or avoided altogether.

PROTEINS AND FATS FOR STABLE BLOOD SUGAR

Proteins and fats have minimal direct impact on blood sugar levels. However, they play essential roles in supporting overall health and promoting satiety, which can help control cravings and stabilize blood sugar.

- **Healthy Protein Choices:** Opt for lean sources of protein, such as poultry, fish, legumes, tofu, and low-fat dairy. These options can provide essential nutrients without contributing to blood sugar spikes.

- **Beneficial Fats:** Incorporate heart-healthy fats, such as avocados, nuts, seeds, olive oil, and fatty fish, into your diet. These fats can improve insulin sensitivity and help manage blood sugar levels.

PORTION CONTROL AND MEAL TIMING

Portion control is essential for controlling blood sugar levels and keeping a healthy weight. By spreading your meals and snacks throughout the day, you can prevent extreme fluctuations in blood sugar.

- **Balanced Meals:** Prepare balanced meals with a variety of proteins, carbohydrates, and healthy fats. This balance can help slow down the absorption of glucose and provide sustained energy.

- **Mindful Eating:** Watch your portions and pay attention to your body's feelings of fullness and hunger signals. Avoid overeating, as large meals can cause rapid spikes in blood sugar.

- **Regular Eating Schedule:** Establishing a consistent eating routine can help stabilize blood sugar levels and improve overall glycemic control.

By incorporating these principles into your daily dietary habits, you can take significant steps toward better blood sugar management. In the next chapter, we will delve into specific foods that are beneficial for those with Type 2 diabetes, guiding you toward creating a diabetes-friendly pantry and meal plan that supports your health and well-being. Remember, small changes can yield significant results, and with dedication and persistence, you can empower yourself to take control of your diabetes journey.

CHAPTER 2

FOODS TO EMBRACE

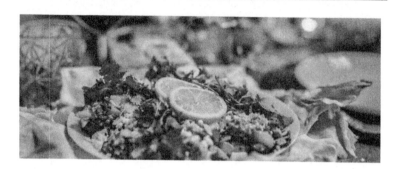

In this chapter, we will explore a variety of wholesome and nutritious foods that can be beneficial for individuals with Type 2 diabetes. These foods are rich in essential nutrients, have a lower impact on blood sugar levels, and can support your overall health and well-being. Let's dive into the types of foods you should embrace in your diabetes-friendly diet.

NON-STARCHY VEGETABLES

Non-starchy vegetables are packed with vitamins, minerals, and dietary fiber, making them an excellent addition to your meals. They have a low glycemic index, meaning they cause minimal spikes in blood sugar levels.

Some examples of non-starchy vegetables include:

- ❖ **Leafy greens:** Spinach, kale, arugula, collard greens, and Swiss chard.
- ❖ **Cruciferous vegetables:** They include cauliflower, Brussels sprouts, Broccoli and cabbage.
- ❖ **Colorful veggies:** Bell peppers, tomatoes, carrots, and eggplants.
- ❖ **Other options:** Zucchini, cucumber, asparagus, mushrooms, and green beans.

Feel free to enjoy these vegetables in various forms, such as raw, steamed, roasted, or stir-fried, to add both taste and nutrients to your meals.

LEAN PROTEINS

Lean proteins are essential for building and repairing tissues, maintaining muscle mass, and regulating blood sugar levels. Including lean proteins in your diet can help you feel full and satisfied without causing significant fluctuations in blood sugar.

Some healthy sources of lean proteins include:

- ❖ **Poultry:** The regular chicken and turkey (without the skin).
- ❖ **Fish:** Salmon, trout, tuna, mackerel, and sardines.
- ❖ **Plant-based proteins**: Tofu, tempeh, edamame, and lentils.
- ❖ **Legumes:** Chickpeas, black beans, kidney beans, and navy beans.
- ❖ **Low-fat dairy** such as cottage cheese, greek yogurt, and skim milk.

Be mindful of portion sizes and preparation methods, aiming for grilled, baked, or broiled options to minimize added fats and calories.

HEALTHY FATS

Contrary to popular belief, fats are an essential part of a balanced diet, even for individuals with Type 2 diabetes. Healthy fats can improve insulin sensitivity, support heart health, and provide a feeling of fullness.

Also, the following healthy fats should be included in your diet as well:

❖ **Avocado:** Rich in monounsaturated fats and fiber.
❖ **Nuts and seeds** such as walnuts, chia seeds, almonds, flaxseeds, and pumpkin seeds.
❖ **Olive oil:** Extra-virgin olive oil is an excellent choice for cooking and dressing salads.
❖ **Fatty fish:** Salmon, mackerel, and trout are rich in omega-3 fatty acids.

While healthy fats are helpful, they are high in calories, thus portion control is crucial.

WHOLE GRAINS AND FIBER-RICH FOODS

Choosing whole grains over refined grains can help stabilize blood sugar levels and provide sustained energy.

Whole grains are higher in fiber, which slows down the absorption of glucose.

Incorporate these whole grains into your diet:

❖ Brown rice
❖ Quinoa
❖ Whole wheat
❖ Barley
❖ Oats
❖ Bulgur
❖ Farro

Additionally, fiber-rich foods such as fruits, vegetables, and legumes can further support your blood sugar management and digestive health.

LOW-GLYCEMIC FRUITS

Fruits contain natural sugars, and while some can cause rapid spikes in blood sugar, others have a lower glycemic index, making them more suitable for individuals with Type 2 diabetes.

Some low-glycemic fruits include:

❖ Berries: Strawberries, blueberries, raspberries, and blackberries.
❖ Cherries
❖ Apples
❖ Pears
❖ Oranges

Remember to enjoy fruits in moderation and opt for whole fruits over fruit juices, as they contain more fiber and have a lower glycemic impact.

Embracing these foods in your diet can provide a wealth of health benefits and help you maintain stable blood sugar levels. In the next chapter, we will discuss the types of foods to limit or avoid, as they can negatively impact blood sugar control and overall health. By making informed choices and building a balanced and diverse diet, you are taking significant steps toward managing your Type 2 diabetes effectively.

CHAPTER 3

FOODS TO LIMIT OR AVOID

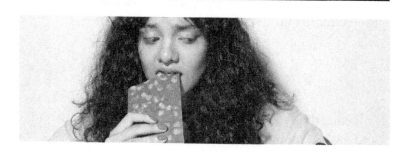

In this chapter, we will explore the types of foods that can negatively impact blood sugar levels and overall health for individuals with Type 2 diabetes. While it's essential to embrace diabetes-friendly foods, being aware of the foods to limit or avoid can further support your efforts in maintaining stable blood sugar levels.

SUGARY AND PROCESSED FOODS

Sugary and processed foods are major culprits when it comes to rapid spikes in blood sugar levels. These foods contain refined sugars and often lack essential nutrients, leading to empty calories that can disrupt glucose control.

Foods to limit or avoid include:

➢ **Soda and sugary beverages**

> **Candy and sweets**
> **Baked goods** (cakes, cookies, pastries)
> **Processed snacks** (chips, crackers)
> **Sweetened breakfast cereals**

Instead of these sugary options, opt for naturally sweetened fruits in moderation and whole, unprocessed foods that provide more nutritional value.

REFINED CARBOHYDRATES

Refined carbohydrates are grains whose exterior bran and germ have been removed, leaving just the starchy endosperm. This process removes essential nutrients and fiber, resulting in quicker absorption and higher blood sugar spikes.

Foods containing refined carbohydrates to limit or avoid include:

> White bread and white rice
> Pasta made from refined flour
> White flour-based baked goods
> Breakfast cereals with added sugars

Instead, choose whole grains like brown rice, quinoa, and whole wheat bread, which contain more fiber and nutrients and have a lower impact on blood sugar.

TRANS FATS AND SATURATED FATS

Trans fats and saturated fats can contribute to insulin resistance and inflammation, increasing the risk of heart disease and impairing blood sugar control.

Foods high in trans fats and saturated fats to limit or avoid include:

➢ Processed and fried foods
➢ High-fat dairy products (eg. full-fat milk, butter, cheese)
➢ Fatty cuts of red meat
➢ Packaged snacks with hydrogenated oils

Opt for healthier fat options like monounsaturated and polyunsaturated fats found in avocados, nuts, seeds, and fatty fish.

HIGH-SODIUM FOODS

High-sodium foods can lead to hypertension and increase the risk of cardiovascular issues, which may complicate diabetes management.

Foods high in sodium to limit or avoid include:

➢ Processed and packaged foods
➢ Canned soups and broths
➢ Deli meats and sausages
➢ Condiments with added salt

Choose fresh or minimally processed foods and use herbs and spices to add flavor instead of relying on excessive salt.

By being mindful of these foods and making informed choices, you can improve your blood sugar control and overall health. It's essential to strike a balance and occasionally enjoy treats in moderation, but the foundation of your diet should consist of diabetes-friendly foods that nourish your body and promote well-being. In the next chapter, we will delve into the art of meal planning and provide sample menus to help you create balanced and delicious meals that support your Type 2 diabetes management journey.

CHAPTER 4

MEAL PLANNING AND SAMPLE MENUS

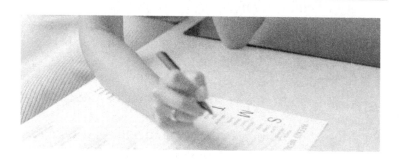

Meal planning is a crucial aspect of managing Type 2 diabetes effectively. By creating well-balanced and nutritious meals, you can regulate blood sugar levels, improve energy levels, and support overall health. In this chapter, we will guide you through the art of meal planning and provide sample menus to help you get started on your journey to better diabetes management.

CREATING BALANCED AND NUTRITIOUS MEALS

When planning your meals, aim to create balanced plates that include a combination of carbohydrates, proteins, and healthy fats. The key is to choose nutrient-dense foods that will provide sustained energy and avoid drastic fluctuations in blood sugar levels.

Here's a general guideline for building balanced meals:

- ❖ Fill one-half of your serving dish with non-starchy veggies like leafy greens, broccoli, and peppers.
- ❖ Reserve a quarter of your plate for lean proteins, like grilled chicken, tofu, or fish.
- ❖ The remaining quarter can be dedicated to whole grains or other healthy carbohydrates, such as brown rice, quinoa, or sweet potatoes.
- ❖ Incorporate a small serving of healthy fats, such as a drizzle of olive oil or a sprinkle of nuts or seeds.

Don't forget to drink lots of water during the day to stay hydrated. Water can help control blood sugar levels and support overall bodily functions.

SAMPLE BREAKFAST, LUNCH, AND DINNER MENUS

To provide a clearer picture of how to build balanced meals, let's explore sample menus for breakfast, lunch, and dinner:

a) Breakfast Menu:
- ❖ Scrambled eggs with spinach and cherry tomatoes (protein and non-starchy vegetables).
- ❖ Whole-grain toast (carbohydrate) topped with mashed avocado (healthy fat).
- ❖ A side of fresh berries (low-glycemic fruit) for a touch of sweetness.

b) Lunch Menu:

❖ Grilled chicken salad with mixed greens (protein and non-starchy vegetables).

❖ Quinoa (whole grain) as a side.

❖ Dressing made with olive oil, lemon juice, and herbs (healthy fat).

❖ A small piece of dark chocolate (in moderation) for dessert.

c) Dinner Menu:

❖ Baked salmon (protein and healthy fats) seasoned with herbs and lemon.

❖ Steamed broccoli and cauliflower (non-starchy vegetables) on the side.

❖ Brown rice (whole grain) or a small portion of sweet potatoes (carbohydrate).

These sample menus demonstrate how to incorporate a variety of foods into your meals, ensuring that you receive essential nutrients while maintaining stable blood sugar levels.

SNACK IDEAS FOR BLOOD SUGAR CONTROL

Choosing diabetes-friendly snacks between meals can help prevent extreme hunger and avoid unhealthy food choices. Below are a couple of delicious and nutritious snack ideas:

❖ Greek yogurt with a handful of nuts (unsalted) and a sprinkle of cinnamon.

❖ Sliced cucumber or carrot sticks with hummus for dipping.
❖ A small apple or a handful of berries paired with a few slices of low-fat cheese.
❖ A boiled egg with a few whole-grain crackers.

Remember to consider portion sizes and the timing of snacks to complement your meals and maintain steady blood sugar levels.

By incorporating balanced and nutritious meals into your daily routine, you can take significant steps toward better managing your Type 2 diabetes. Experiment with different foods, flavors, and cooking methods to find what works best for you. In the next chapter, we will delve into the importance of smart grocery shopping and provide tips for selecting diabetes-friendly options that support your health and well-being.

CHAPTER 5

THE FOOD LIST

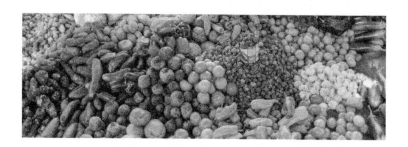

Here's a comprehensive food list for individuals with Type 2 diabetes. The list includes various food categories with examples of diabetes-friendly options within each category:

1. Non-Starchy Vegetables:
- ❖ Spinach
- ❖ Broccoli
- ❖ Cauliflower
- ❖ Brussels sprouts
- ❖ Asparagus
- ❖ Green beans
- ❖ Bell peppers
- ❖ Zucchini
- ❖ Cabbage
- ❖ Cucumbers

2. Leafy Greens:
- ❖ Kale

- ❖ Swiss chard
- ❖ Collard greens
- ❖ Romaine lettuce
- ❖ Arugula
- ❖ Watercress
- ❖ Mustard greens
- ❖ Bok choy
- ❖ Spinach

3. Lean Proteins:
- ❖ Chicken breast (skinless)
- ❖ Turkey breast (skinless)
- ❖ Fish (salmon, trout, cod, tilapia)
- ❖ Shellfish (shrimp, crab, lobster)
- ❖ Lean beef (sirloin, tenderloin)
- ❖ Lean pork (loin chops)
- ❖ Tofu
- ❖ Tempeh
- ❖ Eggs (preferably omega-3 enriched)
- ❖ Low-fat Greek yogurt

4. Whole Grains:
- ❖ Quinoa
- ❖ Brown rice
- ❖ Bulgur
- ❖ Barley
- ❖ Whole wheat pasta
- ❖ Oats (steel-cut or rolled)
- ❖ Farro
- ❖ Millet
- ❖ Buckwheat

5. Legumes:

- ❖ Chickpeas
- ❖ Lentils
- ❖ Black beans
- ❖ Kidney beans
- ❖ Pinto beans
- ❖ Navy beans
- ❖ Black-eyed peas
- ❖ Split peas

6. Healthy Fats:
- ❖ Avocado
- ❖ Olive oil (extra-virgin)
- ❖ Nuts (almonds, walnuts, pistachios)
- ❖ Seeds (flaxseeds, chia seeds)
- ❖ Natural nut butter (almond, peanut, cashew)
- ❖ Fatty fish (salmon, mackerel, sardines)

7. Low-Glycemic Fruits:
- ❖ Berries (blueberries, strawberries, raspberries)
- ❖ Cherries
- ❖ Apples
- ❖ Pears
- ❖ Plums
- ❖ Peaches
- ❖ Oranges
- ❖ Grapefruit

8. Dairy (low-fat or non-fat):
- ❖ Milk
- ❖ Yogurt (plain, unsweetened)
- ❖ Cottage cheese
- ❖ Ricotta cheese
- ❖ Low-fat cheese (mozzarella, feta)

9. Herbs and Spices (for flavor):
❖ Basil
❖ Cilantro
❖ Rosemary
❖ Thyme
❖ Turmeric
❖ Cinnamon
❖ Ginger
❖ Garlic
❖ Paprika

10. Beverages:
❖ Water (plain or infused with citrus or berries)
❖ Herbal teas (unsweetened)
❖ Green tea (unsweetened)

Remember that portion control and overall dietary balance are essential for managing Type 2 diabetes. Always consult with a registered dietitian or healthcare provider to develop a personalized meal plan that fits your individual needs and health goals.

CHAPTER 6

SMART GROCERY SHOPPING FOR TYPE 2 DIABETES

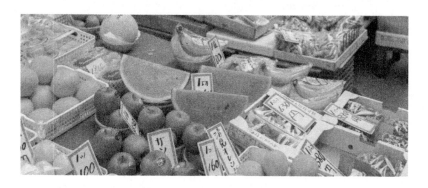

Grocery shopping plays a crucial role in shaping your diet and managing Type 2 diabetes effectively. Making informed choices while navigating the aisles can lead to a well-stocked pantry full of diabetes-friendly options. In this chapter, we will guide you through the process of smart grocery shopping, helping you select nutritious foods that support your blood sugar control and overall health.

READING FOOD LABELS

One of the essential skills for smart grocery shopping is understanding how to read food labels. Labels provide valuable information about the nutritional content of products, allowing you to make informed decisions.

Here are some fundamental tips for interpreting product labels:

❖ Pay attention to the serving size: Ensure you understand the portion size listed on the label and adjust the nutritional values accordingly.

❖ Check the total carbohydrates: Focus on the total carbohydrates and the breakdown of dietary fiber and sugars. Look for products with higher fiber content and lower added sugars.

❖ Be mindful of sodium: Excess sodium can lead to hypertension, so choose products with lower sodium levels.

❖ Look for healthy fats: Opt for products with unsaturated fats, like those found in nuts, seeds, avocados, and fish, rather than trans fats or saturated fats.

TIPS FOR HEALTHY GROCERY SHOPPING

When heading to the grocery store, consider the following tips to make the most of your shopping experience:

❖ **Plan ahead:** Before going to the store, create a shopping list based on your meal plan for the week. This will assist you in remaining focused while avoiding impulse purchases.

❖ **Shop the perimeter:** The outer aisles of the grocery store often contain fresh produce, lean proteins, and dairy products. Focus on filling your cart with items from these sections to build a nutritious foundation for your meals.

❖ **Choose whole, unprocessed foods:** Fresh fruits, vegetables, lean meats, fish, whole grains, nuts, and seeds should be staples in your cart.

❖ **Avoid the center aisles**: The center aisles typically house processed and packaged foods that are high in sugar, sodium, and unhealthy fats. Limit your time in these aisles to minimize exposure to unhealthy options.

❖ **Buy in bulk and freeze:** Purchasing items in bulk can save you money, and freezing extras can help you manage portion sizes and reduce food waste.

BUDGET-FRIENDLY CHOICES

Eating healthily doesn't have to break the bank. Here are some low-cost options to take into account:

❖ **Purchase seasonal produce:** Seasonal fruits and vegetables are frequently less expensive and more flavorful.

❖ **Opt for frozen or canned options:** Frozen and canned fruits and vegetables can be just as nutritious as fresh ones and may be more cost-effective.

❖ **Choose whole grains in bulk:** Purchasing whole grains like brown rice, quinoa, or oats in bulk can be cost-efficient.

❖ **Look for sales and discounts**: Keep an eye out for sales and discounts on healthy items to save money.

By becoming a savvy grocery shopper, you can create a well-rounded and diabetes-friendly pantry, making it easier to stick to your meal plan and maintain stable blood sugar levels.

In the next chapter, we will explore the art of cooking and meal preparation, providing you with tips and techniques to create delicious and diabetes-friendly meals at home. Cooking can be a rewarding experience, allowing you to take control of your diet and health. Let's embark on this culinary journey together!

CHAPTER 7

COOKING AND MEAL PREPARATION

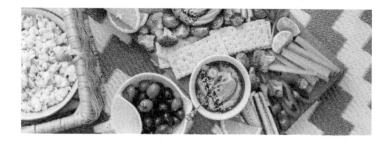

Cooking and meal preparation are essential skills for managing Type 2 diabetes and maintaining a diabetes-friendly diet. By preparing your meals at home, you have greater control over the ingredients and portion sizes, allowing you to create delicious and nutritious dishes that support your blood sugar control and overall health. In this chapter, we will explore the art of cooking and provide you with tips and techniques to make meal preparation a rewarding and enjoyable experience.

HEALTHY COOKING METHODS

Choosing the right cooking methods can significantly impact the nutritional content of your meals.Consider the following healthy cooking methods:

❖ **Grilling:** Grilling is a great way to add flavor to lean proteins and vegetables without adding excess fats. Use marinades with herbs and spices for added taste.
❖ **Baking:** Baking is a low-fat cooking method that can be used for lean meats, fish, and vegetables. Avoid adding excessive oils or butter.
❖ **Steaming:** Steaming preserves the nutrients in vegetables and allows them to retain their natural flavors. Steamed vegetables make a great side dish for any meal.
❖ **Stir-frying:** Stir-frying is a quick and easy way to cook vegetables and lean proteins using minimal oil. Use vegetable broth or a small amount of healthy oil, such as olive oil.
❖ **Boiling:** Boiling is ideal for cooking whole grains, legumes, and pasta. Be sure not to overcook, as this can lead to a higher glycemic impact.

MEAL PREPPING FOR BUSY DAYS

Meal prepping can be a game-changer for individuals with busy schedules. By dedicating time to plan and prepare meals in advance, you can avoid impulsive and unhealthy food choices during hectic moments.

Here are some meal prepping tips:

❖ **Plan your meals for the week:** Create a meal plan for breakfast, lunch, dinner, and snacks, and make a grocery list accordingly.

❖ **Batch cooking:** Prepare larger portions of meals and store them in individual containers for quick and easy access throughout the week.

❖ **Pre-cut and wash vegetables:** Wash, chop, and store vegetables in the refrigerator for quick additions to your meals.

❖ **Make use of versatile ingredients:** - Choose ingredients that can be utilised in several dishes throughout the course of the week. For example, a batch of grilled chicken can be used in salads, wraps, and stir-fries.

❖ **Portion control:** Use food containers with appropriate portion sizes to avoid overeating.

HEALTHY RECIPE MODIFICATIONS

Adapting recipes to make them diabetes-friendly can be both creative and satisfying. Consider making the following modifications to traditional recipes:

- ❖ **Reduce added sugars**: Use natural sweeteners like stevia, monk fruit, or small amounts of honey or maple syrup instead of refined sugar.
- ❖ **Choose whole grains**: Substitute refined grains with whole grains like quinoa, brown rice, or whole wheat flour in recipes.
- ❖ **Trim unhealthy fats:** Use healthier fats, like avocado oil or olive oil, instead of butter or vegetable shortening.
- ❖ **Boost fiber content:** Add vegetables, legumes, or seeds to recipes to increase the fiber content and slow down the absorption of glucose.

COOKING RESOURCES

Take advantage of cooking resources to expand your culinary skills and discover new diabetes-friendly recipes:

- ❖ **Diabetes-friendly cookbooks:** Look for cookbooks specifically designed for individuals with diabetes. They often provide nutritional information and helpful tips.
- ❖ **Online recipe websites:** Explore reputable websites that offer a wide range of diabetes-friendly recipes.
- ❖ **Cooking classes:** Consider attending cooking classes or workshops that focus on healthy and diabetes-friendly cooking techniques.
- ❖ **Social media:** Follow diabetes-friendly food bloggers and chefs on social media for inspiration and recipe ideas.

BONUS CHAPTER 1

NUTRITIOUS FAMILY-FRIENDLY RECIPES

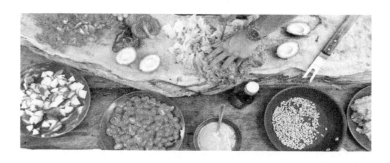

Here are ten delicious and nutritious family-friendly recipes that cater to the dietary needs of individuals with diabetes while appealing to everyone in the household. These recipes will make mealtimes enjoyable for the whole family:

1. Grilled Chicken Fajita Bowls:

Ingredients:
- ❖ One pound boneless, skinless chicken breasts, thinly sliced
- ❖ 1 red bell pepper, sliced
- ❖ 1 green bell pepper, sliced
- ❖ 1 yellow bell pepper, sliced
- ❖ 1 onion, sliced
- ❖ 2 tablespoons olive oil

- ❖ 1 tablespoon chili powder
- ❖ 1 teaspoon cumin
- ❖ 1/2 teaspoon paprika
- ❖ Salt and pepper to taste
- ❖ Brown rice or cauliflower rice (to be used for a low-carb option)
- ❖ Toppings: Guacamole, salsa, shredded lettuce, chopped tomatoes, and plain Greek yogurt (as a sour cream substitute)

Instructions:
1. In a bowl, mix the olive oil, chili powder, cumin, paprika, salt, and pepper. Toss in the sliced chicken until uniformly coated. Marinate for 20-30 minutes.
2. Toss in the sliced chicken until uniformly coated. Grill the chicken until cooked through and slightly charred. Remove from heat and set aside.
3. In the same grill or grill pan, cook the sliced bell peppers and onions until tender and slightly charred.
4. Serve the grilled chicken and veggies over a bed of brown rice or cauliflower rice. Top with your choice of toppings, and enjoy the family-friendly fajita bowls together.

2. Baked Salmon with Lemon-Dill Sauce:

Ingredients:
- ❖ 4 salmon fillets
- ❖ 2 tablespoons olive oil
- ❖ 1 lemon, sliced
- ❖ 2 tablespoons fresh dill, chopped
- ❖ Salt and pepper to taste

❖ **Lemon-Dill Sauce:** Mix 1/2 cup plain Greek yogurt, 1 tablespoon fresh dill, 1 tablespoon lemon juice, 1 teaspoon lemon zest, and a pinch of salt.

Instructions:
1. Preheat the oven to 375°F (190°C). Line a baking sheet with parchment paper and arrange the salmon fillets on it.
2. Drizzle olive oil over the salmon, then season with salt and pepper. Place lemon slices on top of each fillet.
3. Bake the salmon for 12-15 minutes or until it flakes easily with a fork.
4. Serve the baked salmon with the lemon-dill sauce on the side. Pair it with a side of steamed vegetables and quinoa for a complete family meal.

3. Vegetable Stir-Fry with Tofu:

Ingredients:
❖ 1 block of firm tofu, cubed
❖ 2 tablespoons soy sauce (low-sodium)
❖ 1 tablespoon sesame oil
❖ 2 tablespoons olive oil
❖ 2 cloves garlic, minced
❖ 1 tablespoon fresh ginger, minced
❖ 1 red bell pepper, sliced
❖ 1 cup broccoli florets
❖ 1 cup snap peas
❖ 1 carrot, thinly sliced
❖ 2 green onions, chopped
❖ Sesame seeds for garnish

Instructions:
1. In a bowl, marinate the tofu cubes in soy sauce and sesame oil for 15-20 minutes.
2. Heat up the olive oil in a big skillet or wok over a medium-high temperature. Add the marinated tofu and cook until crispy and golden brown. Remove the tofu from the skillet & place it aside.
3. In the same skillet, add more olive oil if needed, and sauté garlic and ginger until fragrant.
4. Add the sliced bell pepper, broccoli, snap peas, and carrot to the skillet. Stir-fry until the vegetables are tender-crisp.
5. Return the crispy tofu to the skillet, toss everything together, and cook for another minute.
6. Serve the vegetable stir-fry with tofu over steamed brown rice or quinoa. Garnish with sesame seeds and chopped green onions to finish.

4. Turkey and Black Bean Chili:

Ingredients:
- ❖ 1 lb ground turkey (lean)
- ❖ 1 onion, diced
- ❖ 2 cloves garlic, minced
- ❖ 1 red bell pepper, diced
- ❖ 1 can (14 oz) diced tomatoes (no added sugar)
- ❖ 1 can (14 oz) black beans, drained and rinsed
- ❖ One cup chicken or veggie broth (low sodium)
- ❖ 2 tablespoons chili powder
- ❖ 1 teaspoon cumin
- ❖ 1/2 teaspoon paprika
- ❖ Salt and pepper to taste

❖ Optional toppings: Avocado slices, chopped cilantro, and shredded cheese (in moderation)

Instructions:
1. First, brown the ground turkey over a medium-high heat in a Dutch oven or large pot.
2. Add the diced onion, minced garlic, and diced red bell pepper to the pot. Sauté until the vegetables are softened.
3. Stir in the diced tomatoes, black beans, chicken or vegetable broth, chili powder, cumin, paprika, salt, and pepper.
4. Bring the chili to a boil, then reduce the heat and let it simmer for about 20-25 minutes, allowing the flavors to meld.
5. Serve the turkey and black bean chili hot, and top with optional toppings as desired.

5. Veggie and Chicken Skewers with Yogurt-Dill Dip:

Ingredients:
❖ One pound of boneless, skinless chicken breast (cut into cubes)
❖ Cherry tomatoes
❖ Bell pepper chunks (various colors)
❖ Red onion chunks
❖ Zucchini slices
❖ Olive oil
❖ Salt and pepper to taste
❖ Wooden or metal skewers

❖ Yogurt-Dill Dip: Mix 1 cup plain Greek yogurt, 1 tablespoon fresh dill, 1 tablespoon lemon juice, 1 teaspoon lemon zest, 1 clove minced garlic, and a pinch of salt.

Instructions:
1. Start by preheating the grill or grill pan to medium-high temperature.
2. Assemble the chicken and vegetable chunks onto the skewers, alternating between chicken, tomatoes, bell pepper, red onion, and zucchini.
3. Drizzle olive oil over the skewers and season with salt and pepper.
4. Grill the skewers for about 10-12 minutes, turning occasionally until the chicken is cooked through and the vegetables are tender.
5. Serve the veggie and chicken skewers with the yogurt-dill dip on the side. Add a side salad or quinoa for a complete family-friendly meal.

6. Spaghetti Squash Bolognese:

Ingredients:
❖ 1 large spaghetti squash
❖ 1 lb lean ground beef (or turkey)
❖ 1 onion, finely chopped
❖ 2 cloves garlic, minced
❖ 1 can (14 oz) crushed tomatoes (no added sugar)
❖ 1 tablespoon tomato paste
❖ 1 teaspoon dried oregano
❖ 1 teaspoon dried basil
❖ Salt and pepper to taste

- ❖ Grated Parmesan cheese (in moderation) for garnish
- ❖ Fresh basil leaves for garnish

Instructions:
1. First, preheat the oven to 400°F (200°C), then cut it in half lengthwise & remove the seeds from the spaghetti squash .
2. Place the spaghetti squash halves cut-side down on a baking sheet. Bake for 30-40 minutes or until the squash is tender and can be easily shredded with a fork.
3. In a large skillet, cook the ground beef (or turkey) over medium heat until browned. Drain any excess fat.
4. Add the chopped onion and minced garlic to the skillet and sauté until softened.
5. Stir in the crushed tomatoes, tomato paste, dried oregano, dried basil, salt, and pepper. Next, don't forget to simmer for 10 to15 minutes so that the flavors can meld.
6. Once the spaghetti squash is cooked, use a fork to shred the flesh into spaghetti-like strands.
7. Serve the Bolognese sauce over the spaghetti squash, garnish with grated Parmesan cheese and fresh basil leaves, and enjoy this tasty and low-carb alternative to traditional spaghetti.

7. Veggie-Packed Mini Frittatas:

Ingredients:
- ❖ 6 large eggs
- ❖ 1/4 cup milk (low-fat or unsweetened almond milk)
- ❖ 1 cup chopped spinach
- ❖ 1/2 cup diced bell peppers (various colors)

- ❖ 1/4 cup diced tomatoes
- ❖ 1/4 cup diced onions
- ❖ 1/4 cup shredded low-fat cheddar cheese
- ❖ Salt and pepper to taste

Instructions:
1. Preheat the oven to 375°F (190°C). Grease a muffin tin or use silicone muffin cups.
2. In a bowl, whisk together eggs, milk, salt, and pepper until well combined.
3. Add chopped spinach, diced bell peppers, tomatoes, onions, and shredded cheddar cheese to the egg mixture. Stir until evenly distributed.
4. Pour the mixture into the muffin cups, filling each cup about two-thirds full.
5. Bake for 20-25 minutes or until the frittatas are set and slightly golden on top.
6. Allow the mini frittatas to cool slightly before serving. They can be refrigerated and enjoyed as quick and portable breakfast options throughout the week.

8. Turkey and Vegetable Sloppy Joes:

Ingredients:
- ❖ 1 lb ground turkey
- ❖ 1 onion, finely chopped
- ❖ 2 cloves garlic, minced
- ❖ One cup of diced bell peppers (should be of various colors)
- ❖ 1 cup grated carrots
- ❖ 1 can (14 oz) crushed tomatoes (no added sugar)
- ❖ 2 tablespoons tomato paste

- 1 tablespoon Worcestershire sauce
- 1 tablespoon apple cider vinegar
- 1 tablespoon honey or a sugar substitute (optional, adjust to taste)
- Salt and pepper to taste
- Whole grain hamburger buns (or lettuce wraps for a low-carb option)

Instructions:
1. In a large skillet, cook the ground turkey over medium heat until browned. Drain any excess fat.
2. Add the chopped onion and minced garlic to the skillet and sauté until softened.
3. Stir in the diced bell peppers and grated carrots, after that cook for a few minutes until you can see the vegetables are tender.
4. Add the crushed tomatoes, tomato paste, Worcestershire sauce, apple cider vinegar, honey (or sugar substitute), salt, and pepper. Simmer for 10-15 minutes, allowing the flavors to meld.
5. Serve the turkey and vegetable mixture on whole grain hamburger buns or lettuce wraps. Enjoy these healthier and flavorful Sloppy Joes with your family.

9. Stuffed Bell Peppers:

Ingredients:
- 4 large bell peppers (various colors)
- 1 lb lean ground beef (or turkey)
- 1 cup cooked quinoa (or brown rice)
- 1 cup diced tomatoes
- 1 cup black beans (canned, drained, and rinsed)

- ❖ 1 cup chopped spinach
- ❖ 1/2 cup diced onions
- ❖ 2 cloves garlic, minced
- ❖ 1 tablespoon chili powder
- ❖ 1 teaspoon cumin
- ❖ Salt and pepper to taste
- ❖ Shredded low-fat cheddar cheese (in moderation) for topping

Instructions:

1. Preheat the oven to 375°F (190°C) then remove the tops of the bell peppers and discard the seeds and membranes.
2. In a large skillet, cook the ground beef (or turkey) over medium heat until browned. Drain any excess fat.
3. Add the diced tomatoes, black beans, chopped spinach, diced onions, minced garlic, chili powder, cumin, salt, and pepper to the skillet. After that, cook(while stirring occasionally) until the vegetables are tender.
4. Stir in the cooked quinoa (or brown rice) and mix everything together.
5. Stuff each bell pepper with the mixture and place them in a baking dish.
6. Bake the stuffed bell peppers for 20-25 minutes, or until the peppers are tender.
7. Sprinkle shredded low-fat cheddar cheese on top of each stuffed bell pepper and return them to the oven for a few more minutes until the cheese is melted.
8. Serve the stuffed bell peppers as a wholesome and colorful meal the whole family will enjoy.

10. Banana-Oat Blender Pancakes:

Ingredients:
- ❖ 2 ripe bananas
- ❖ 2 large eggs
- ❖ 1 cup rolled oats
- ❖ 1/2 cup unsweetened almond milk (or any milk of choice)
- ❖ 1 teaspoon baking powder
- ❖ 1/2 teaspoon vanilla extract
- ❖ Pinch of cinnamon (optional)
- ❖ Fresh berries and sugar-free syrup for topping

Instructions:
1. In a blender, combine the ripe bananas, large eggs, rolled oats, unsweetened almond milk, baking powder, vanilla extract, and a pinch of cinnamon (if using). Blend until smooth.
2. Preheat a non-stick skillet or griddle over medium heat. Lightly coat the surface with cooking spray or a small amount of oil.
3. Pour the pancake batter onto the skillet, using about 1/4 cup of batter for each pancake.
4. Cook the pancakes for 2-3 minutes on each side, or until bubbles form on the surface and the edges are slightly set.
5. Flip the pancakes and cook for an additional 1-2 minutes until golden brown.
6. Serve the banana-oat blender pancakes with fresh berries and sugar-free syrup for a delicious and wholesome breakfast that the whole family will love.

These additional family-friendly recipes offer a variety of flavors and textures, making mealtime enjoyable for everyone in the household. Remember to adjust the recipes according to your dietary preferences and health needs. With these tasty and diabetes-friendly recipes, you can promote a healthy lifestyle for your family and foster a love for nutritious and delicious food. Happy cooking and bon appétit!

These family-friendly recipes are designed to be delicious, healthy, and easy to prepare, making them suitable for all members of the household. Whether you have diabetes or not, the whole family can enjoy these flavorful meals together, fostering a sense of togetherness around the dinner table.

Encourage your loved ones to embark on a journey of wellness and make positive dietary choices that support overall health. Remember that modifying recipes to suit individual dietary needs is always an option. Embrace the joy of cooking and savor the bond that sharing nutritious and delicious meals can create among family members.

Happy cooking and bon appétit!

CHAPTER 8

DINING OUT WITH TYPE 2 DIABETES

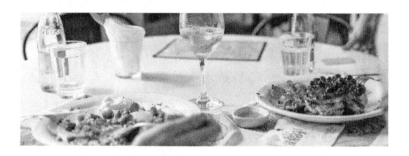

Dining out can be a delightful experience, but it can also present challenges for individuals with Type 2 diabetes. Navigating restaurant menus and making healthy choices while eating out is essential for maintaining stable blood sugar levels and supporting your diabetes management goals. In this chapter, we will explore strategies to dine out with confidence, ensuring that you make informed decisions and enjoy your meals without compromising your health.

MAKING HEALTHIER CHOICES AT RESTAURANTS

When dining out, there are several tips you can follow to make healthier choices:

a) **First of all, check the menu ahead of time:** Many restaurants have their menus online already. Take the time to review the menu beforehand, so you can plan ahead and choose diabetes-friendly options.

b) **Focus on non-starchy vegetables:** Opt for dishes that include a variety of non-starchy vegetables. Salads, grilled vegetables, and vegetable stir-fries can be excellent choices.

c) **Choose lean proteins:** Look for dishes with lean proteins like grilled chicken, fish, or tofu. Avoid fried or breaded options.

d) **Request modifications:** Don't be afraid to ask the server to make adjustments to your meal. For instance, ask for sauces or dressings on the side to control portions and avoid added sugars.

e) **Control portions:** Restaurant portions are often larger than necessary. Consider splitting a meal with a dining partner or ask for a to-go box to save part of the meal for later.

NAVIGATING FAST FOOD OPTIONS

While fast food restaurants may not be the ideal choice for individuals with Type 2 diabetes, there are ways to make healthier choices if you find yourself at a fast-food establishment:

❖ **Look for grilled options:** Many fast food chains offer grilled chicken or fish sandwiches that can be a better choice than fried items.

❖ **Choose salads wisely:** Opt for salads with plenty of vegetables, lean protein, and a vinaigrette dressing on the side. Avoid salads with fried toppings and high-calorie dressings.

❖ **Skip the sugary beverages:** Choose water, unsweetened tea, or diet drinks instead of sugary sodas and fruit-flavored beverages.

❖ **Limit sides and extras:** Avoid supersizing or adding high-calorie sides to your meal. Stick to smaller portions or skip the extras altogether.

STAYING MINDFUL OF HIDDEN SUGARS AND CARBOHYDRATES

When dining out, it's essential to be mindful of hidden sugars and carbohydrates in sauces, dressings, and condiments. Some menu items may seem healthy but can be loaded with added sugars and unhealthy fats.

❖ **Opt for homemade dressings**: Request dressings or sauces made with natural ingredients and minimal added sugars.

❖ **Be cautious with condiments**: Use condiments sparingly or ask for them on the side to control the amount you consume.

❖ **Choose wisely:** Some seemingly healthy menu items may contain hidden sugars or high-carb ingredients. Read the descriptions carefully, and when in doubt, ask your server about the ingredients.

MANAGING SPECIAL OCCASIONS

During special occasions or celebratory events, you may find yourself faced with more indulgent food choices. It's essential to strike a balance and enjoy these moments without compromising your diabetes management.

1. **Plan ahead:** If you know you'll be attending a special event, eat balanced meals earlier in the day to help offset any indulgences.
2. **Watch portion sizes:** Enjoy smaller portions of indulgent foods to satisfy your taste buds without overindulging.
3. **Control your environment:** Offer to bring a diabetes-friendly dish to the gathering, ensuring that there's something healthy and delicious for you to enjoy.

By being proactive and informed when dining out, you can make smart choices and still savor delicious meals while effectively managing your Type 2 diabetes.

In the next chapter, we will discuss the importance of physical activity in diabetes management. Exercise plays a significant role in controlling blood sugar levels, improving insulin sensitivity, and supporting overall well-being. Let's explore the benefits of staying active and how you can incorporate exercise into your daily routine.

BONUS CHAPTER 2

THE ROLE OF PHYSICAL ACTIVITY

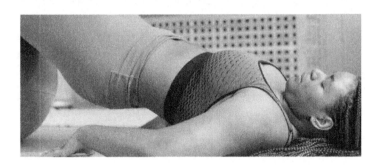

Physical activity is a key component of managing Type 2 diabetes effectively. Regular exercise offers numerous benefits, including improved blood sugar control, increased insulin sensitivity, weight management, and enhanced cardiovascular health. In this chapter, we will explore the importance of physical activity in diabetes management and provide strategies for incorporating exercise into your daily routine.

EXERCISE AND BLOOD SUGAR REGULATION

Engaging in physical activity can help lower blood sugar levels by increasing the uptake of glucose by your muscles, reducing insulin resistance, and improving overall glycemic control. When you exercise, your muscles use glucose for energy, which helps to reduce blood sugar levels.

Types of exercises that are particularly beneficial for blood sugar regulation include:

A. **Aerobic exercises:** Activities like brisk walking, cycling, swimming, dancing, and jogging can help lower blood sugar levels and improve cardiovascular health.
B. **Resistance training:** Strength training exercises, such as weightlifting or using resistance bands, can increase muscle mass and improve insulin sensitivity.
C. **Flexibility and balance exercises:** Activities like yoga and tai chi can help improve flexibility, balance, and overall well-being.

INCORPORATING EXERCISE INTO YOUR ROUTINE

Finding ways to incorporate exercise into your daily routine can make it easier to stick to a regular physical activity regimen. Below are a few suggestions to get yourself started:

❖ **Start gradually:** If you're new to exercise, begin with short and manageable sessions and gradually increase the intensity and duration over time.
❖ **Find activities you enjoy:** Choose exercises that you enjoy doing, as this will increase the likelihood of sticking to your routine.
❖ **Set realistic goals:** Establish achievable exercise goals and celebrate your progress along the way to stay motivated.

❖ **Make it a habit:** Schedule regular exercise sessions into your daily or weekly routine to establish a habit.

FINDING MOTIVATION

Staying motivated to exercise can sometimes be a challenge. These are some pointers to keep you on the right track:

1. **Enlist support:** Exercise with a friend or family member, or join a fitness class or support group to stay motivated and accountable.
2. **Track your progress:** Keep a record of your exercise sessions and monitor your improvements over time. This can help you see the positive impact of your efforts.
3. **Reward yourself:** Treat yourself to small rewards for achieving your exercise goals, such as a relaxing bath, a favorite book, or spending time doing an enjoyable activity.

SAFETY PRECAUTIONS

Before starting any exercise program, it's essential to consult with your healthcare provider, especially if you have any pre-existing health conditions. They can help determine the most suitable exercise plan for your specific needs and ensure your safety.

Below are some precautions to keep in mind to ensure your safety while exercising:

❖ **Warm-up and cool down:** Always warm up before exercising and cool down afterward to prevent injuries and muscle strain.

❖ **Stay hydrated:** To stay hydrated, drink lots of water prior to, during, as well as after exercise.

❖ **Check your blood sugar:** Monitor your blood sugar levels before and after exercise, especially if you take insulin or certain medications that can lower blood sugar.

By incorporating regular physical activity into your life, you can enhance your diabetes management, improve your overall health, and enjoy a more active and fulfilling lifestyle.

In the next chapter, we will discuss the relationship between Type 2 diabetes, weight management, and the strategies you can employ to achieve and maintain a healthy weight. Let's explore the impact of weight on diabetes and how you can approach weight management effectively.

BONUS CHAPTER 3

WEIGHT MANAGEMENT AND TYPE 2 DIABETES

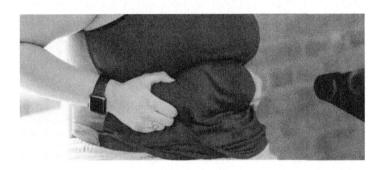

Maintaining a healthy weight is essential for individuals with Type 2 diabetes, as it can significantly impact blood sugar control and overall health. Achieving and sustaining a healthy weight can improve insulin sensitivity, reduce the risk of complications, and enhance your quality of life. In this chapter, we will explore the relationship between weight management and Type 2 diabetes and provide strategies to help you achieve and maintain a healthy weight.

THE LINK BETWEEN WEIGHT AND TYPE 2 DIABETES

Excess weight, particularly around the abdomen, is closely associated with insulin resistance, a key factor in Type 2 diabetes. When your cells become resistant to insulin, it becomes more challenging for glucose to enter your cells, leading to elevated blood sugar levels.

Weight management is essential for diabetes management because losing even a modest amount of weight can have a significant impact on blood sugar control and overall health. It can reduce the need for diabetes medications, improve cholesterol and blood pressure levels, and lower the risk of cardiovascular complications.

SETTING REALISTIC WEIGHT LOSS GOALS

When embarking on a weight loss journey, it's crucial to set realistic and achievable goals. Focusing on small, incremental changes can lead to long-term success and prevent feelings of frustration or disappointment.

Here are some pointers for creating realistic weight loss targets:

❖ Aim for gradual weight loss: Losing about 1-2 pounds per week is a realistic and sustainable target.
❖ Break your goals into smaller milestones: Set smaller, achievable targets along the way to stay motivated and track your progress effectively.
❖ Focus on overall health: Instead of solely fixating on the scale, prioritize improving your overall health through a balanced diet and regular exercise.

STRATEGIES FOR HEALTHY WEIGHT MANAGEMENT

Adopting a combination of healthy eating, regular physical activity, and lifestyle changes can support your weight management efforts:

1. **Balanced diet:** Focus on a balanced diet that includes a variety of nutrient-dense foods, such as non-starchy vegetables, lean proteins, whole grains, and healthy fats. Be mindful of portion sizes and avoid excessive sugar and unhealthy fats.
2. **Regular exercise:** Engage in regular physical activity, aiming for at least 150 minutes of moderate-intensity aerobic exercise per week, along with muscle-strengthening activities on two or more days per week.
3. **Stay consistent:** Make healthy eating and exercise a part of your daily routine. Always remember that the key to obtaining and maintaining a healthy weight is consistency, that's just it.
4. **Manage stress:** Chronic stress can lead to emotional eating and hinder weight management efforts. Stress-reduction practises such as yoga, mindfulness, or meditation should be used.
5. **Get enough sleep:** Lack of sleep can disrupt hunger hormones and lead to unhealthy food choices. Each night, always aim for 7-9 hours of good, uninterrupted sleep.

SEEKING PROFESSIONAL SUPPORT

If you find it challenging to manage your weight on your own, consider seeking support from healthcare professionals or a registered dietitian specializing in diabetes management. They can provide personalized guidance and create a tailored plan that fits your needs and lifestyle.

Remember that achieving a healthy weight and maintaining it is a journey, not a quick fix. Be patient with yourself and celebrate every small achievement along the way. By focusing on your overall health and well-being, you can take significant strides in managing your Type 2 diabetes and embracing a healthier and more fulfilling life.

In the final chapter, we will conclude our journey through "Type 2 Diabetes Food List" by summarizing the key takeaways and offering a message of empowerment and hope as you continue your diabetes management journey. Let's reflect on what we've learned and the positive impact you can make in your life.

CHAPTER 9

FREQUENTLY ASKED QUESTIONS (FAQS)

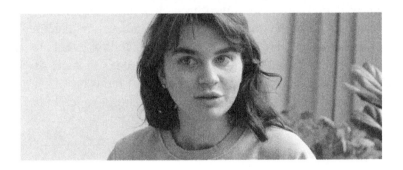

Throughout our journey exploring "Type 2 Diabetes Food List," you might have come across questions about diabetes management, dietary choices, and lifestyle adjustments. In this chapter, we address some frequently asked questions to provide further clarity and support on your path to better diabetes management.

Q1: Is it possible to completely eliminate sugar from my diet?

While it's not necessary to completely eliminate sugar from your diet, it's essential to be mindful of your sugar intake. Natural sugars found in fruits and some dairy products are acceptable in moderation. However, added sugars, particularly in processed and sugary foods, should be limited or avoided, as they can lead to blood sugar spikes and impact overall health negatively.

Q2: How do I handle social situations and special events while managing my diabetes?

Social events and special occasions can present challenges, but with planning and mindfulness, you can enjoy these moments without compromising your diabetes management. Consider eating a healthy meal before attending events to avoid excessive indulgence. When faced with an array of food options, choose smaller portions and focus on diabetes-friendly choices, such as non-starchy vegetables and lean proteins.

Q3: Are there specific fruits I should avoid?

While fruits are a healthy part of a balanced diet, some fruits have higher sugar content and may cause rapid spikes in blood sugar levels. Fruits such as watermelon and pineapple have higher glycemic indices, so it's advisable to consume them in moderation. Instead, prioritize lower-glycemic fruits like berries, apples, and pears.

Q4: Can I still enjoy alcoholic beverages with Type 2 diabetes?

Alcoholic beverages can affect blood sugar levels, so moderation is essential. It's best to limit alcohol intake and avoid sugary cocktails and sweetened alcoholic beverages.

Instead, opt for moderate amounts of dry wine, light beer, or distilled spirits mixed with sugar-free mixers. Always monitor your blood sugar when consuming alcohol and drink responsibly.

Q5: How can I remain motivated to exercise on a regular basis?

Staying motivated to exercise can be challenging, but finding activities you enjoy and setting achievable goals can help. Consider exercising with a friend or enrolling in a fitness class for additional motivation and accountability. Tracking your progress and celebrating your achievements, no matter how small, can keep you motivated and committed to regular physical activity.

Q6: Can I still eat out at restaurants while managing my diabetes?

Yes, of course you can eat out at restaurants while even managing your diabetes. When dining out, review the menu in advance and choose diabetes-friendly options like non-starchy vegetables, lean proteins, and whole grains. Request modifications to suit your dietary needs, such as sauces on the side or smaller portion sizes.

Q7: Should I follow a specific diet plan for diabetes management?

There is no one-size-fits-all diet plan for diabetes management. It's essential to work with a registered dietitian or healthcare provider to create a personalized meal plan that considers your specific health needs and lifestyle. Concentrate on a well-balanced diet consisting of nutrient-dense foods and reasonable portion sizes.

Q8: Can I reverse Type 2 diabetes through lifestyle changes?

In some cases, making significant lifestyle changes, such as adopting a healthy diet, regular exercise, and weight management, can lead to significant improvements in blood sugar control and potentially reverse Type 2 diabetes. However, this depends on individual factors, and it's crucial to work closely with healthcare professionals to monitor and manage your condition effectively.

Remember that every individual's experience with Type 2 diabetes is unique, and it's essential to address any concerns or questions you may have with your healthcare team. Armed with knowledge and determination, you can successfully manage your Type 2 diabetes, make positive lifestyle changes, and lead a fulfilling life filled with good health and well-being.

CONCLUSION

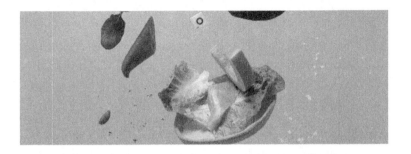

In "Type 2 Diabetes Food List," we have embarked on a comprehensive journey to empower individuals with Type 2 diabetes to take charge of their health and well-being. Throughout this book, we have explored the fundamental principles of a diabetes-friendly diet, meal planning strategies, and the role of physical activity in managing blood sugar levels effectively.

Armed with knowledge, practical tips, and a positive mindset, you can make informed choices about your diet, create balanced and delicious meals, and engage in regular physical activity to support your diabetes management goals. While living with Type 2 diabetes may present challenges, know that you are not alone on this journey.

Remember the key takeaways from this book:

1) **Embrace a Balanced Diet:** Prioritize non-starchy vegetables, lean proteins, whole grains, and healthy fats in your meals. Be mindful of portion sizes and limit added sugars and unhealthy fats.

2) **Plan and Prepare:** Meal planning and preparation can set you up for success. Embrace meal prepping, try new recipes, and experiment with different flavors and cuisines.

3) **Stay Active:** Regular physical activity is essential for blood sugar control, weight management, and overall well-being. Find activities you enjoy and make exercise a regular part of your routine.

4) **Seek Support and Knowledge:** Reach out to healthcare professionals, registered dietitians, and support groups for guidance and encouragement. Stay up to date with the treatment of diabetes and the newest research.

5) **Celebrate Progress:** Acknowledge and celebrate your achievements, no matter how small. Every positive step you take contributes to better diabetes management and a healthier life.

As you continue your diabetes management journey, remember that you have the power to make a positive impact on your health. Be patient with yourself, practice self-compassion, and never lose sight of hope.

Diabetes management is a lifelong commitment, but with determination, discipline, and a positive outlook, you can thrive and live a fulfilling life with Type 2 diabetes. Take each day as an opportunity to make healthy choices, and remember that every step you take towards better health is a testament to your strength and resilience.

May this book serve as a valuable guide and source of inspiration as you navigate your path to optimal diabetes management. Embrace the power within you, and know that you have the tools to lead a vibrant and healthy life, living well with Type 2 diabetes.

Wishing you health, happiness, and a bright future ahead!

My Little Request

Thank You For Reading This Book!
I really appreciate all of your feedback and
I love to hear what you have to say.

I need your input to make the next version of this
book and my future books better.

Please take two minutes now to leave a helpful review on
Amazon letting me know what you thought of the book:
Thanks so much!
- Bell Quintana

Attribution

All images used in this book were downloaded from *pexels.com.*

NOTES

Printed in Great Britain
by Amazon

45811035R00046